To My Readers

Be sure to write to me at my e-mail address, jimhewittwriting@aol.com. When I receive your e-mail, I will add you to my SPECIAL e-mail list. This group of readers will receive updates on any already published subject matter. Also any time I publish a new book they will know about it in advance.

Titles by James Hewitt

Sick Building Syndrome

The Christmas Tree

Ramblings

The Adirondack Cookbook

Memory: Lost & Found

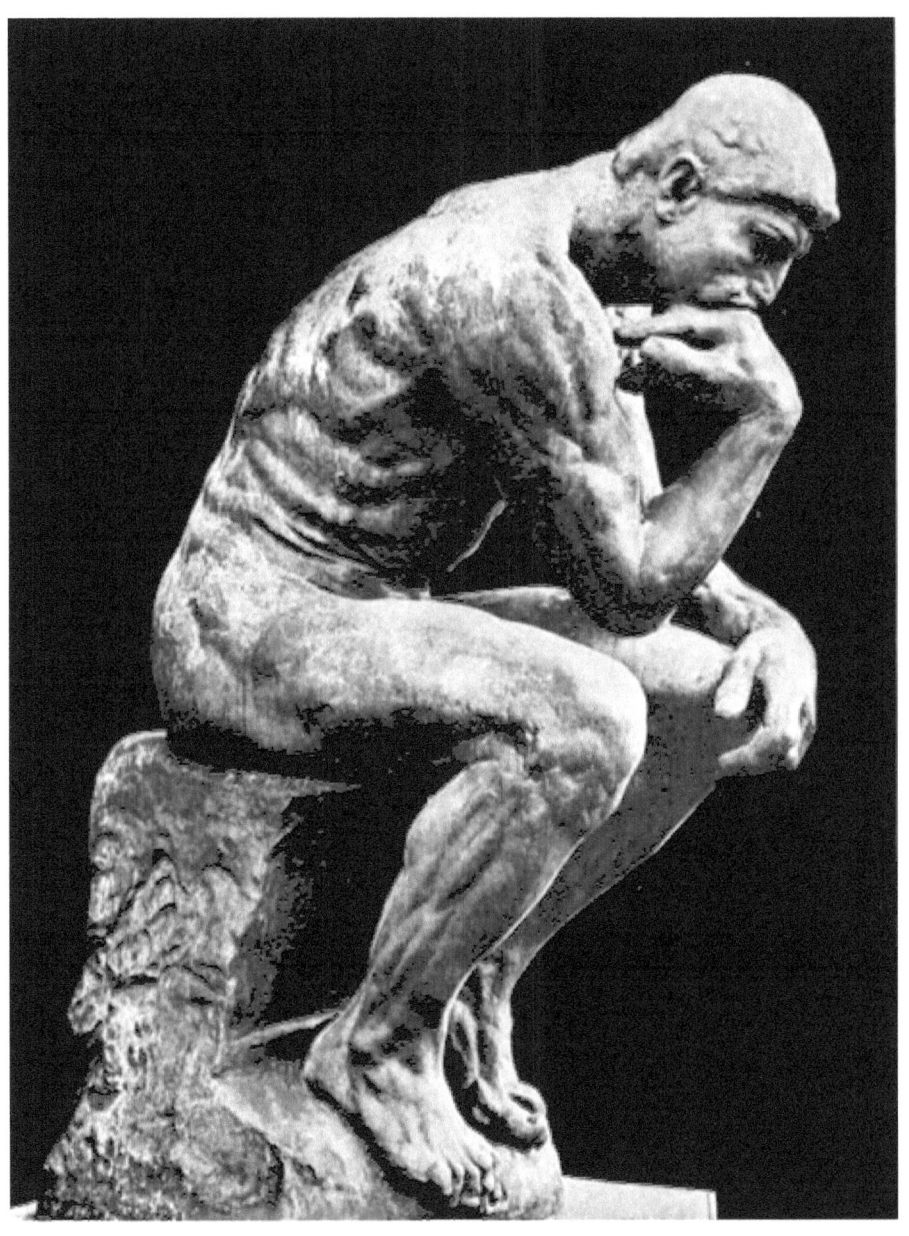

James Hewitt RN

ISBN: 978-1-4357-1757-2

GNU Free Documentation License

Published by Lulu Distribution (www.lulu.com)

Printed in the USA.

Thanks

For my Mother, Rose Ann Hewitt, who has always been my number ONE supporter. It is true what they say about a Mothers' Love. Her memory is as sharp as a tack.

Thanks to my Wife, Virginia Anne Hewitt for all her extra support. Thanks for being patient with all my long hours of research and quirky phrases. She is definitely my better half. She is my light in the darkness.

Thanks to all the folks who helped me by reviewing my facts and information.

Dedication

This book is dedicated to all the families and people affected by a Memory Disorder. The three most common forms of dementia are; Alzheimer's disease, multi-infarct dementia (MID) or vascular dementia, and Lewy body dementia.

An estimated 2 million people in the United States suffer from severe dementia. Another 1 to 5 million people experience mild to moderate dementia. Five to eight percent of people over the age of 65 have some form of dementia and that number doubles every 5 years over age 65.

A portion of the proceeds from every book sold will go toward sponsoring research to help prevent and treat memory disorders.

Table of Contents

Introduction

It seems like ever since I hit my early 40s, my memory has been in a state of rebellion. I can remember all the big things in my life, like my name, the date, my family, and so forth. It's the little things like my wife asking me to pick up milk on the way home that I forget. I often tell people, "I am too young to be acting this old".

In this book, I will educate the reader regarding memory loss and its prevention. This book will be split into three easily read sections. The first section will talk about memory. The second section in the book will educate the reader about memory loss and how it can happen. Finally in the third and final section I will discuss some methods to improve memory. In this section I will also mention the nutritional aspect of memory.

As an added bonus, I have included a section on nutritional supplements and their claims to memory improvement. I do not recommend any specific supplement. I have included this section for your information only.

The results of any of the treatments or use of any solutions in this book can be both positive and negative in different people, depending upon the particular facts and circumstances regarding the person's age, health, medical history, and physical condition. In the medical field, everyone should be treated differently, and on an individual basis. The treatments suggested here will not ensure successful treatment in every situation, but they can be helpful.

I firmly recommend consulting your family Physician, before trying any of the supplements in the bonus section. Many natural supplements can interact with prescribed medications.

The Human Brain

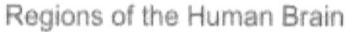

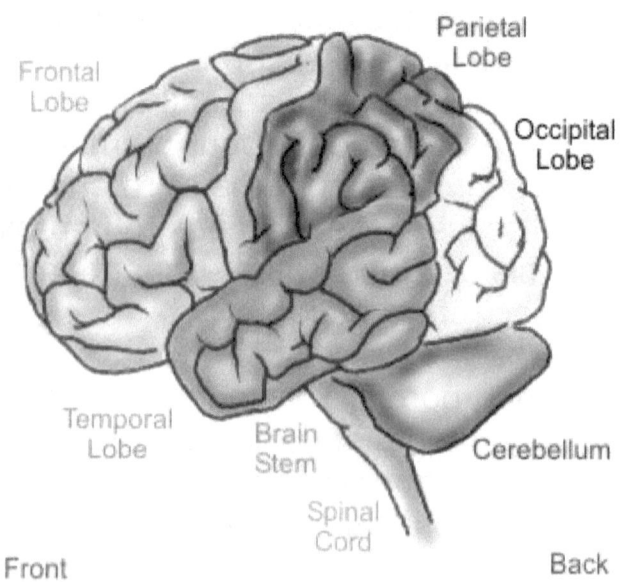

www.science.ca/images/Brain_Witelson.jpg

The language and information provided in this book is primarily intended for the use by the non-medical person. This book has been written with a very minimal amount of medical terminology and jargon. My goal has been to create a book that will educate anyone without them needing an encyclopedia and dictionary to make sense of the contents of this book. This book is designed for use as an educational product for the regular person.

Please do keep in mind however, that medical situations are often complex and that this book is not a substitute for good clinical judgment and consultation with an experienced Physician.

Have you ever wondered whether your memory lapses are normal or a sign of more serious problems? This book will hopefully expand your horizons.

Memory

When we learn, we organize, shape, and strengthen our brains. Human beings are a constantly learning machine. From the day we are born our brains are ready to capture our experiences and encode them into a web of nerve connections. Our brains are the engines that drive the human learning machines. A hundred billion or more nerve cells are crammed into three pounds of complex tissue inside our skull, that we refer to as the brain. It is amazing to think that this three pounds runs our bodies processes and thoughts.

The brain is an amazing control center for the human body. It is responsible for controlling our movement, language, hearing, vision, coordination, smell and memory. It is efficient in quickly and precisely relaying correct messages to and from the brain and body.

Why do we experience changes in our mental abilities as we age? What happens in our brains to cause these changes? What can we do to keep our minds sharp? Are there any tricks to improve our memory? I hope to answer these questions for you as you read this book.

Brain fitness for people of all ages has gone beyond the "use it or lose it" viewpoint. I prefer to the more optimistic viewpoint of "use it, to improve it!" As long as we are alive, our mind will never stop learning.

Before I begin to delve into the mind and memory, I first must dispense with some memory myths. The first is that you can't change your brain. The old adage that you cannot teach an old dog new tricks is wrong. Your brain is constantly changing in response to your experiences. Everything we do and think about is reflected in the patterns of activity in our brains. Scientists can see these patterns in brain-imaging scans like an electroencephalogram (EEG) that shows which parts of the brain are functioning during specific tasks.

An EEG is a diagnostic tool used to image the brain while it is performing a cognitive task. This allows Doctors to detect the location and magnitude of brain activity involved in the various types of human cognitive functions. An EEG allows us to view and record the changes in our brain activity during the time we are performing the task. Images are acquired by using electrodes to monitor the amount of electrical activity at different points on our scalp. EEGs are non-invasive and do not involve any X-rays, radiation, or injections. EEGs have been used for many years and are considered very safe.

Another myth is that memory decline is inevitable as we age. Many people reach very old age and are still sharp as ever. Genetics clearly plays a role in "successful aging," but how we live our lives on a day-to-day basis is also critical.

The brain doesn't make new brain cells is another myth. This myth was widely believed for generations, but has recently been proven false. Scientists now know that certain areas in the brain, such as the hippocampus, where new memories are created and the olfactory bulb, which is the scent processing center regularly generate new brain cells.

The last myth I plan to dispel is that we lose brain cells every day and eventually just run out. Most regions of the brain do not lose brain cells as you age. You may lose some nerve connections. It's also possible that you can even grow new brain cells and create new connections, or prevent the ones you have from withering, if you exercise your brain. You will read up on this in the third part of the book, called <u>Methods to Improve Memory</u>.

Whether or not certain events or information is retained in memory is dependent upon an individual's love for the subject matter and it's dramatic, emotional, auditory, and visual impact. A great example of this is how effortlessly it is to remember the scenes of an engrossing movie for a long time.

On the other hand it takes a concerted effort to memorize dry irrelevant data on a page, which usually results only in short recall. It is through the use of lengthy, repetitive study of written words, many schools attempt to coerce students to force information for lengthy recall.

A College Professor I had once said, "Remembering is just thinking." No pun intended, but I cannot remember his name. A sign that my memory needs some work.

The ability to richly re-experience autobiographical memory is thought to be unique to humans and is important for advanced decision making and our quality of life. A person who loses this ability to recall personal episodic memories as a result of a memory disorder or serious brain injury can be tremendously devastating to the individual and their family.

I will try to explain how a memory occurs. I will touch on our nervous system briefly, so that you can have an understanding of its complexity. There are volumes of books about the human nervous system. I will try to keep the medical jargon down to a minimum.

First I will have to examine our neurological system. What is it? What are its components? Why and how does it work? All are great questions, so jump right in and have some fun.

What is it? The Neurological System is the human bodies information processor. What are its components? What do the parts do for the body?

The Neurological System is divided into two major parts. They are the Central Nervous System (CNS) and the Peripheral Nervous System (PNS). The Central Nervous System is the body's information headquarters, which ultimately regulates all of the bodies functions. The CNS consists of the brain and spinal cord. The PNS is responsible for the remainder of the body. It includes the cranial nerves, spinal nerves, and all the major sense organs.

The PNS is the major player when it comes to regulating your body. It is composed of the Somatic

Nervous System (SNS) and Autonomic Nervous System (ANS). The SNS is responsible for all voluntary muscular activities. The ANS is responsible for all activities that occur automatically and involuntarily, such as breathing and your heartbeat.

Great, now that we have covered some basics let us get into the good stuff. The good stuff is our neural network. The network in question is that squishy gray ball of neurons known as brain cells. Each of us has approximately 100 billion at birth. Every neuron is connected to others through many threadlike parts called axons and a smaller number of cordlike parts called dendrites. The number of these connections among brain cells is well into the trillions. The number of patterns that are possible in a network of trillions, is infinite.

By now you have ascertained that the system used in forming a memory is a complex system. You are still most likely confused as to how your memories get formed. Information flows from the outside world through our sight, hearing smelling, tasting and touch sensors. Our mind stores for fractions of a second the sensory information in areas located throughout our cortex. Some data is moved into short-term memory. Some of that information also goes into long term storage in various parts of the cortex.

When our mind recalls a memory it re-fires many of the same neural paths that were used originally to sense the experience. Our mind therefore re-creates the event.

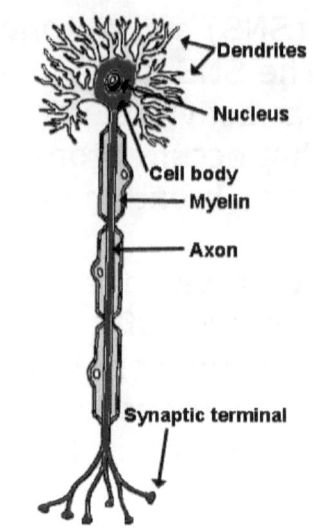

www.indiancowboy.net

Modern medical society has three generally accepted classifications of memory. These classifications are based on the duration of memory retention. The three distinct types of memory are sensory memory, short term memory and long term memory. I will explain what each type entails and their importance.

Here is a picture to help show where in our mind our senses and short term memory occur.

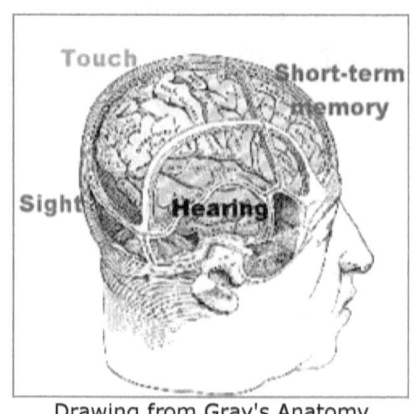

Drawing from Gray's Anatomy

So, what is sensory memory? According to Ecyclopedia.com, sensory memory, "is the very short-term memory store for information being processed by the sense organs".   Sounds great, but what does it really mean? Sensory memory takes place approximately during the initial 200 - 500 milliseconds after an item has been perceived by one of our five senses. Sensory memory is the ability to look at an item, and remember what it looked like with just a second of observation. Memorization, is an example of sensory memory. This type of memory cannot be prolonged via rehearsal. Sensory memory allow us to take a 'snapshot' of our environment, and to store this information for a short period.

Short term memory is best defined by Ecyclopedia.com, as "a memory system capable of holding a limited amount of information for brief periods, up to a maximum of about 20 or 30 seconds, although it can be renewed indefinitely if the information within it is rehearsed". Some information that is processed by our sensory memory can be transferred to short term memory. Our short term memory allows one to recall something from several seconds to as long as a minute without rehearsal. This capacity is very limited.

Long term memory can store much larger quantities of information for potentially unlimited duration, sometimes even for our whole life span. It is defined by Encyclopedia.com as, "A type of memory containing information that is stored for periods ranging from about 30 seconds to many decades".

Below is a picture of the spine courtesy of Cedars Mt. Sinai.

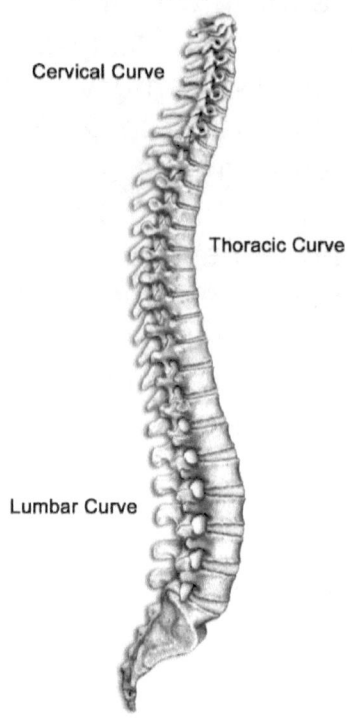

www.cedars-sinai.edu

Illnesses of the Mind

Brain disorders account for one-third of all chronic illnesses. Brain diseases affect millions upon millions of people in the U.S.. and they affect not only those with chronic illnesses, but also their families, friends, and colleagues. Unfortunately, there are many illnesses related to the mind. I am concentrating on Memory Disorders.

Brain disorders, like stroke or head injury, are most commonly the result of damage to brain tissues. Other brain-related disorders are caused by progressive failure and death of nerve cells. This is known as "neurodegeneration". It occurs in Alzheimer's and Parkinson's diseases. A sad part of aging is that as we age, our brain becomes more vulnerable to many brain disorders, and may be affected by health problems elsewhere in the body.

When is memory loss not so normal? Amnesia, which is the loss of memory, is not a part of the normal aging process. While it may take longer to learn new information or to recall learned information, with a little time and extra effort memory occurs. Some people are more forgetful, but this might be because of health conditions. Some health conditions that can affect memory are depression, heart disease, thyroid disease, vitamin deficiencies, or medication side effects.

The physical signs of some chronic illnesses begin gradually, and may not be noticeable for years. Symptoms may be mild or severe, frequent or infrequent, or they may not be evident at all on a day-to-day basis. Living with a chronic condition can pose enormous challenges, physically, emotionally, and financially. Your illness doesn't have to control you.

Here is a list of items to do when confronted by a chronic illness. Learning to accept and cope with the fact that you need to make these adjustments is part of the process of managing your illness.

1. Understand your illness
2. Get the right medical care
3. Monitor your health
4. Eat well and exercise
5. Take care of your Mental Health
6. Adjust your lifestyle
7. Get plenty of sleep
8. Join a support group

Understanding how and why brain functions change as we grow older may lead to new therapies and medications that could slow, stop, or prevent these processes altogether. Changes vary greatly from one person to the next, and may include the following, depending on their medical and psychological history. As a person ages brain mass shrinks, the brains outer surface thins, our white matter decreases, and the brains chemical messengers decrease.

Memory loss is abnormal in people with mild cognitive impairment or dementia, which is the loss of intellectual functions severe enough to interfere with everyday social or occupational functioning.

With mild cognitive impairment it is important to remember that memory impairments occur without loss of independent functioning. People can be forgetfulness and struggle while performing self-care tasks, but they still are able to do so without the direct help of another person.

Dementia occurs when a person's memory, language, and cognition are so impaired that self-care tasks can no longer be performed without assistance from another person. A person cannot perform complex daily tasks, such as remembering to pay bills or take medications. There is a loss of insight and an awareness of the memory loss. The person will demonstrate poor judgment and may even exhibit behavioral symptoms, like irritability, worrying, anger, agitation, and even paranoia.

You may be wondering, "How did my neurological system become so unbalanced?" It does not take much to affect our overall health. The fact of the matter is that chronic health conditions do not just "happen." There can be a genetic component that predisposes someone to becoming chronically ill, but research has shown that there are other factors often within our control that are usually the cause.

These controllable factors that cause a person to have an unhealthy neurological system may be caused by poor diet, chronic infections, acute infections, pesticides, stress, heavy metal exposure, and toxicity.

Vitamin, mineral, and amino acid deficiencies affect the neurological system's ability to function effectively. This may lead to certain levels of neurological impairment such as mental confusion, loss of concentration, depression and anxiety.

Chronic and Acute Infections are a big factor that can cause neurologic impairments. Candida yeast may be responsible for a variety of neurological symptoms, including Brain Fog and Depression. This is directly related to the enormous amounts of toxins that this fungus emits. Syphilis can invade the central nervous system and may cause neurological impairment and stroke-like symptoms. Bacterial and viral meningitis, which is inflammation of the tissues surrounding the spinal cord and the brain can cause confusion.

Brain Fog involves a persistent or episodic cognitive dysfunction, and may be associated with forgetfulness, confusion, slowed thinking, distractibility, depersonalization, and the inability to remember the correct words when speaking or writing. Brain fog is so named because the sufferer can feel like a cloud literally surrounds them that reduces the speed at which things can be recognized or clearly seen.

A study conducted on vineyard workers showed that long term, low-level exposures to pesticides have measurable effects on cognition.

Chronic stress and negative thinking can wreak havoc on the neurological system. Chronic stress can trigger mental disorders such as anxiety and depression.

Heavy metals such as aluminum, lead, and mercury accumulate in the brain. Ongoing studies are examining possible links between high levels of toxic metals and severe neurological disorders such as Alzheimer's Disease.

I have previously mentioned the three types of memory, but what is memory? Memory is "The power or process of reproducing or recalling what has been learned and retained", according to Merriam Webster Dictionary. Our ability to remember and to recall our past is what links us to our families, to our friends, to our community. Take a moment and think of something funny. Now think about a cherished thought. Now image how you would feel not having either of those two memories.

As a person ages, subtle changes in memory occur, sometimes unnoticed, but at other times these changes can be disturbing to ourselves or those around us. Most of our normal changes in memory and cognition are of little importance, as they do not interfere with our daily activities or our quality of life. It is only when the memory loss prevents us from performing daily tasks and living in our accustomed roles in life that the loss, becomes a health concern that needs further evaluation by a health care professional.

As we age slight changes occur in our cognition that affect memory. Simple forgetfulness, such as forgetting where you put your eye glasses or the slowing in recalling names, dates, and events can be part of the normal process of aging. Memory might be affected differently by aging. Everyone has preserved memory functions that enable us to perform tasks, such as eating. We also have the ability to recall general knowledge, like how a telephone works or how to open a door. Unfortunately, as we age we have declining memory functions. We have slight difficulty learning new information. It generally takes longer to learn something new and to be able to recall it.

Nutritionally there are foods that we should try to avoid to help our memory. We should AVOID foods that can hinder the neurological system, like alcohol, caffeine, refined sugars, artificial sweeteners, nitrates, deep fried foods, and partially hydrogenated oils.

Alcohol impairs brain function and motor skills. Caffeinated beverages such as coffee, tea, and soft drinks can over stimulate the neurological system. Avoid energy drinks that contain extra caffeine and sugar that over stimulate the neurological system. Refined sugars that may contribute to Candida yeast overgrowth, which I mentioned earlier in this section. Artificial sweeteners such as Aspartame and Splenda® can have toxic effects on the neurological system.

Nitrites are found in processed foods, such as hot dogs, lunch meats, and bacon. Some studies have shown that children who eat hot dogs more than two times a week have a higher risk of brain tumors and brain cancers. Partially hydrogenated oils are found in many processed baked goods and snack foods. Deep fried food, fast food, and junk food, many which contain trans fats should also be avoided or consumed in limited portions.

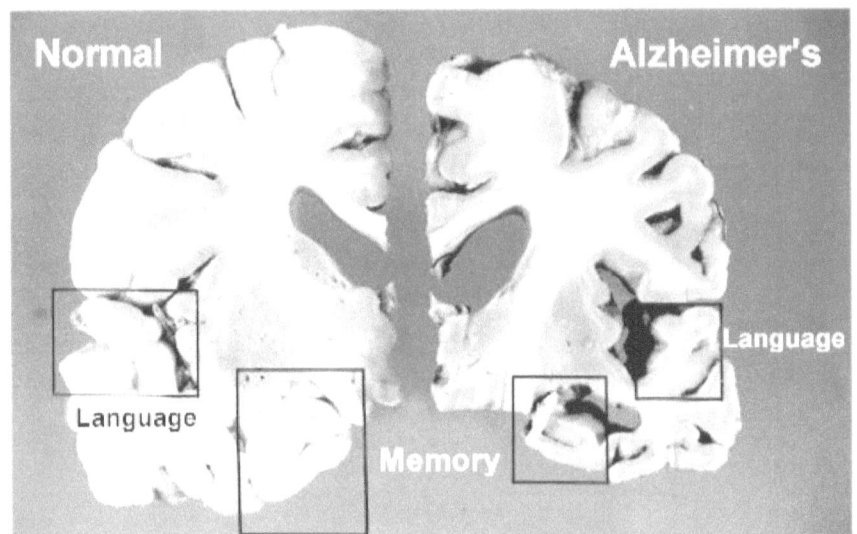

www.umsl.edu

    This picture gives a comparison of a normal brain versus a brain affected by Alzheimer's disease. The Alzheimer's brain is severely atrophied. Language and memory have significant decreases in size.

Methods to Improve Memory

At this point, you are probably scratching your head wondering, can normal memory be preserved during the aging process? The answer is, Absolutely, Yes! Keeping your mind active and your memory sharp is a key part of aging well and enjoying better quality of life as you grow older. By challenging and engaging your brain, and learning throughout your life, you can help maintain your healthy brain. As a Registered Nurse, I am often amazed at how young and vital a senior citizen can be as long as they have stayed active and healthy.

Our brain is the most extraordinary and complex creation in the universe, so it is worth feeding, nurturing, and being offered stimulating challenges. Your brain works much better than you might think. It is capable of making a huge and even better "unlimited" number of synaptic connections. Thinking can be hard work and humans by nature tend to do as little thinking as possible. Sometimes thinking feels like lifting weights, that's why people usually pick the first solution that comes to mind without making further efforts to find alternative better solutions.

In order for you to stay mentally fit you need to do mental stimulation. Brain games can provide that stimulation through challenges. Studies have shown that doing puzzles, playing games or simply learning a new language can build neural networks in the brain. There is an association between keeping cognitively active and a decreased risk of Alzheimer's disease.

The best way to benefit from exercise is to participate for 30 minutes each day, instead of spending longs hours just once or twice a week. People tend to benefit more from exercise and mental training if it's done regularly, because we learn new things constantly. These new things need to be stored, retained and retrieved from time to time, otherwise they soon become forgotten.

It's very useful to train your mind on a daily basis, because our brains are composed of different areas of "mental muscles". The mind can be strengthened through mental exercises otherwise they become weak for lack of practice. Memory games or concentration games are very helpful and provide a great training under stressful situations. Memory games also have a long term effect in preventing or delaying mental illnesses, such as Alzheimer.

Research has shown that continued education helps preserve "cognitive reserve" and delays the onset of dementia. A healthy diet lowers the risk of dementia. A person can engage in cognitive training, reasoning training, and speed of process training to improve cognition. It has been shown that playing board games like chess, checkers, cards, puzzles, cross word puzzles, word games, and musical instruments will definitely delay the onset of dementia. Studies have shown that if a person stays socially active the onset of any impairment will be slowed down. Also reducing cardiovascular risks, such as coronary artery disease, hypertension, and high cholesterol, can delay the onset of dementia.

By improving memory, we have to make a distinction between improving the short-term memory and the long-term memory. Improving the short-term memory is relatively easy, the only way we can increase the amount of information we can hold in short-term memory is to group items into more effective chunks.

The first mechanism for good remembering is paying attention. You can't remember what you never noticed. It sounds obvious, but memory problems often start right there. At least mine do as I am absent minded and easily distracted. As a student I would often find myself distracted or daydreaming out a window in class.

The second mechanism is rehearsal, another obvious one. Saying or doing something over and over tends to make it stick. That's how most of us learned the multiplication tables, and it's the method by which a lot of education is conducted. Although it works pretty well, it's cumbersome. A teacher once told me that to remember something it needs to be repeated or rehearsed three times in our minds. For me to remember, I need to read, write, and speak it. This my three ways of rehearsing.

The third mechanism is where it gets interesting. The brain remembers by forming links and slotting new information into existing frameworks. I always remember the that dessert has two letter's s, since for dessert I like two scoops of ice cream. This is where you can work on improving your own memory processing to make sure you'll be able to retrieve a memory later.

Mnemonics is the science of remembering. It's a bag of tricks designed to help a person remember data, especially isolated, minute details. This is the type of information that we have the hardest time holding onto.

Mnemonics relies on linking, clumping, and framing information so it is more easily remembered. Greek orators invented it so they could give speeches without using notes, and people have been refining and expanding their techniques ever since.

There are several ways to improve your long-term memory. A recall for a word pair improves greatly when the two words are connected by an image. Imagery can also be useful in the keyword method of learning. Improving image also depends on the environment. You should try to find a logical link between words when you have to remember them. Therefore you can learn better idiom if they are arranged by theme.

Another way to improve retrieval is to practice. Ask yourself what you are learning. For example, suppose you have two hours to learn a text that can be read through in 30 minutes. It will not be effective to read the text four times. Instead, it will be more effective if you read the text one time. During that reading you select the difficult parts, and then later you return only to the parts that were difficult.

Nutrition plays a big role in your body's health. You can be a marathon runner or a genius but without proper nutrition your body will not perform well if at all. An unhealthy neurological system may be caused by poor diet. There are many vitamin, mineral, and amino acid deficiencies that can affect the neurological system's ability to function effectively. These deficiencies may lead to certain levels of neurological impairment such as mental confusion, loss of concentration, depression and anxiety.

Of all the memory "enhancers" touted today, the simplest may be food. New research shows that eating protein, carbohydrates or fat may boost memory in healthy older people. A study conducted by Randall J. Kaplan of the University of Toronto, found that eating 15 to 60 minutes before engaging in work that requires memory appears to be beneficial for people in their 60s and 70s.

There are many dietary things you can do to support the healthy functioning of your neurological system. Studies have shown that a diet rich in omega-3 fatty oils have lower rates of major depression. You can obtain your omega-3 from different sources. Fish is an important source of omega-3, but you should limit your intake since it may be contaminated with mercury, which I previously mentioned is a neurotoxin. When buying fish choose wild fish rather than farm raised fish. Wild fish obtain omega-3 naturally through their diet. Fish farms, on the other hand, feed their fish land-based foods that may contain little or no omega-3. Some other non-fish food sources of Omega-3 oils are from walnuts and flax meal.

An essential amino acid, tryptophan can be obtained from the diet or through supplementing with tryptophan. Tryptophan helps the body produce serotonin and melatonin which play a role in mood regulation and the quality of a persons sleep. Some foods that contain tryptophan are turkey, beans, whole grain rice, lentils, hazelnuts, sesame seeds, and sunflower seeds.

Saturated fats have a bad reputation, but they are actually essential for fat soluble vitamin delivery to the body, and for a host of other body processes. In fact, 60% of the brain is made up of saturated fat. My wife can honestly say my mind is fat. A good source of saturated fat to add to your diet is organic extra virgin oil and coconut oil.

Iron helps the neurotransmitters essential to memory function properly. Your brain can be sensitive to low amounts of iron. Ask your Medical Doctor at your next appointment to perform a blood test to check your ferritin level, which will reveal even a moderate iron deficiency.

I have heard positive results from people who have played one of the new games specially designed to improve your focus. These games could have the indirect effect of getting your memory in shape. Whenever you solve puzzles or do brainteasers, you're making the connections between your neurons work more efficiently. Your brain is very much like a muscle and it needs constant challenges to grow. The old adage is true, "If you don't use it, you will lose it."

Here are some simple ideas for everyday activities to help with memory. They say pictures are worth a thousand words. To help stimulate memory design a scrapbook of very special memories and review them with your senior citizen often. Put pictures in frames and ad captions of names, dates, and events to help remind them of the important people and dates.

Save all greeting cards and holiday pictures. Re-reading personal letters and viewing pictures can help jog memories. Write notes to remind seniors. If someone is forgetting who you are and they can see well enough, try wearing a name tag like "My name is Jim. You are my Aunt. I love you." This will help them feel less conscious about not being able to remember your name.

For more alert seniors, or those who want to keep memories before they are lost, good reviews are coming in for a handheld game by Nintendo called, Brain Age. Also they can play the children's game Memory. Memory games with a deck of cards can be fun and mentally stimulating. Ask your senior questions about childhood pets, homes, games, and friends. This will help them with their memory recall.

According to a study posted online in the Archives of Neurology, taking an elderly friend or relative out for a fish dinner will help their memory. The old saying that, 'fish is brain food' is true. Eating fish once a week or more was associated with a ten percent per year slower rate of cognitive decline in older people.

To sum it all up, the ways to help keep your mind sharp is to first relax as tension and stress are associated with memory lapses. Managing stress improves memory. Next, you must concentrate and focus on what you are trying to remember. It is important to slow down, because if you are rushing, you may not be focused or paying attention. You must be organized. Always write it down. Repetition improves recall. Try repeating names when meeting new people, or repeating facts when you're learning new information. Last but not least, visualize it. A visual image will help you to remember and improve your recall.

Bonus Section

As a Nurse I just had to read up on the supplements known as, brain boosters or memory enhancers. Patients often ask about vitamins and minerals. After looking into theses widely advertised supplements I made the determination that they are simply brain health herbs with a host of different actions. I found some similarities between the products.

A lot of them are antioxidants, which annihilate free radicals in your body. These free radicals are molecules that cause damage wherever they land. Also many of these supplements are brain feeders that increase oxygen and glucose supply to the brain. Others are neurotransmitter helpers. As previously mentioned in the first section, brain cells communicate through neurotransmitters. Many of these herbs either increase neurotransmitter production or decrease their rate of destruction. Finally, they also fall into a category I call the Neuroprotectors. Neuroprotectors protect nerve cells from damage caused by poor circulation, toxic compounds, and other problems. This is vital, since once a nerve cell is damaged, you can't fix it or grow a new one. Senility unfortunately results from a lifetime of such nerve damage.

These next few listed supplements are sold as brain boosting and/or memory helping pills. Buyer beware. Once again, I reiterate that you consult with your family Physician, before trying any of the supplements in the bonus section. These supplements are not regulated by the United States Food and Drug Administration. Manufacturers do not need to register their products with FDA nor get FDA approval before producing or selling dietary supplements. Many natural supplements can interact with prescribed medications.

When I did a search on the internet, these three supplements popped up everywhere. I reiterate that I do not endorse any of these products. This section is purely for your own information.

Brain Reload - consists of Serine, Choline, DMAE, Alcar, and DLPA.

FOCUS Factor - contains DMAE, a natural substance found in fish, botanical extracts, such as bacopa, huperzine , vinpocetine, and DHA, an important omega-3 fatty acid.

Mind-Power-Rx - contains Ginkgo Biloba leaf extract, Mucuna-Pruriens extract, Ashwagandha extract, Bacopa Monniera extract, Gotu-Kola extract, Reishi extract, Ginseng extract, Fo-Ti extract, and Rhodiola extract.

Here is a list of the supplement ingredients from above and their health related claims.

Alcar (Acetyl-L-Carnitine) - increases acetylcholine levels in the brain, which is one of the main neurotransmitters needed for learning and memory.

Ashwagandha extract - possesses anti-inflammatory, antitumor, anti-stress, antioxidant, hemopoetic, and rejuvenating properties.

Bacopa Monniera extract - used as a therapeutic herb for the treatment of cognitive impairment, thus supporting its possible anti-Alzheimer's properties.

Choline - an essential nutrient for humans that is used to synthesize membrane phospholipids and the neurotransmitter acetylcholine.

DHA - a long chain fatty acid that is a component of complex lipids, including the membranes of the central nervous system.

DLPA - a substance that occurs naturally in the brain and appears to elevate mood.

DMAE - thought to work by increasing production of the neurotransmitter acetylcholine.

Fo-Ti extract - Chinese believe it restores vitality and virility, working especially on the liver and the reproductive, urinary and circulatory systems.

Ginkgo Biloba - reported to maintain peripheral circulation to the arms, legs and brain. Also, Ginkgo is supposed to help improve memory, especially occasional mild memory problems associated with aging.

Ginseng extract - has a sedative effect on the central nervous system and is beneficial for numerous bodily functions.

Gotu-Kola extract - has an ancient reputation for aiding mental clarity and lowering blood pressure.

Huperzine - delays the breakdown of acetylcholine in the brain.

Mucuna-Pruriens extract - supportive role in HGH secretion by helping to build new nerve and brain cells.

Reishi extract - traditional tonic for well being. It has been a remedy in China for thousands of years and is considered an "elixir of life".

Rhodiola extract - used to treat fatigue, depression, anemia, impotence, gastrointestinal aliments, infections and disorders of the nervous system.

Serine - provides nutritional support for brain functions and maintain normal memory.

Vinpocetine - supposed to help keep healthy oxygen flow, nutrient supply, and energy production to the brain

Medical Terminology

Alzheimer's - a progressive form of presenile dementia that is similar to senile dementia except that it usually starts in the 40s or 50s; first symptoms are impaired memory which is followed by impaired thought and speech and finally complete helplessness.

axon - extended part of a neuron that carries an impulse towards the synapse and transmits the message to other neurons.

brain - organ of your body located inside your skull, responsible for everything you think, feel, see, hear, do, and remember.

brainstem - regulates things like heart rate, breathing, swallowing, digestion, blinking, and more.

central nervous system - brain and spinal cord make up the central nervous system.

cerebellum - cerebellum is a busy switching station, by receiving messages from most of the muscles and joints in your body.

cerebral cortex - the largest part of your brain, that does a lot of the brain work, like thinking, decisions, and creativity. It's responsible for the five senses, memory and emotion.

cerebrospinal fluid - clear fluid that fills in all of the spaces between the parts of your brain. It gives the brain a cushion.

corpus callosum - bridge of nerve fibers that connect the two hemispheres of the Cerebral Cortex.

dementia - severe impairment or loss of intellectual capacity and personality integration, due to the loss of or damage to neurons in the brain.

dendrite - branch-like part of a neuron that receives impulses and information from other neurons.

dopamine - neurotransmitter important in helping to regulate physical movement, pleasure, and thought and is missing in patients with Parkinson's Disease.

endorphins - family of neuro-transmitters that help to ease pain and cause sleepiness.

hypothalamus - thumb sized region deep in the middle of the brain that monitors the body's internal functions and helps regulate things like hunger, thirst, body temperature, and hormones.

long term memory - information stored in the brain and retrievable over a long period of time, often over the entire life span of the individual.

medulla oblongata - A part of the brainstem that regulates breathing, heartbeat, and blood flow.

memory - the capacity to recall previously experienced sensations, information, data and ideas.

memory disorder - any diseases, disorders, or medical conditions that affect memory loss.

nerve fiber - axons growing along side each other on their way to other parts of the body or brain.

neuron - the brain is made up nerve cells called neurons. Neurons are the building blocks of your brain. Your brain is estimated to have 100 billion neurons.

neurotransmitters - are the messengers that travel between one brain cell and another. They are chemical signals that neurons use to talk to each other, which is what makes your brain work.

peptides - function as neurotransmitters that often act as helper signals with other neurotransmitters in ways similar to how the endorphins help to regulate the feeling of pain.
peripheral nervous system - nerves that connect your spinal cord to the rest of your body.

remote memory - memory that is serviceable for events long past, but not able to acquire new recollections.

replacement memory - the replacing of one memory with another.

screen memory - a consciously tolerable memory serving to conceal another memory that might be disturbing or emotionally painful if recalled.

serotonin - neurotransmitter that is involved in mood, sleep, mental health, blood pressure and heartbeat.

sensory memory - the ability to retain impressions of sensory information after the original stimulus has ceased.

short-term memory - memory that is lost within a brief period (from a few seconds to a maximum of about 30 minutes) unless reinforced.

spinal cord - carries instructions to the rest of your body. The spinal cord is your body's information superhighway to and from the skin, muscles, and joints.

ventricles - hollow spaces in your brain that are filled with cerebrospinal fluid.

References

American Journal of Clinical Nutrition
Vol. 74, No. 3,
Pages 410-411
September 2001
www.ajcn.org

Anatomy of the Human Body
Henry Gray
Twentieth Edition
Philadelphia: Lea & Febiger, 1918
New York: Bartleby.com, 2000

BrainReload, LLC
4425-C Treat Blvd.
Suite 279
Concord, CA 94521
888-655-0728
www.brainreload.com

Britannica Encyclopedia
331 North La Salle Street
Chicago, IL 60610
www.Britannica.com

Cedars-Sinai Medical Center
8700 Beverly Blvd.
Los Angeles, CA 90048
310-4-CEDARS
www.cedars-sinai.edu

Dictionary.com
www.dictionary.com

eVitamins
6060 Collection Drive
Shelby Twp, MI 48316
888-222-6056
www.evitamins.com

Focus Factor
Vital Basics, Inc.
100 Commercial Street
Suite 200
Portland, Maine 04101
800-825-1423
www.focusfactor.com

GCS Research Society
4692 Quebec St.
Vancouver, BC
V5V 3M1
604-876-5790
www.science.ca

Mind Power RX
212 Technology Drive
Suite B
Irvine, California 92618
877-225-2466
mindpowerrx.com

Morphonix LLC
3001 Bridgeway
Ste K-343
Sausalito, CA 94965
415-331-5010
www.morphonix.com

NeuroHealth
227 Centerville Road
Warwick, RI 02886
401-732-3332
www.neurohealth.info

Prevention Magazine
www.prevention.com

University of Missouri
Saint Louis
866-669-7140
www.umsl.edu

US National Library of Medicine
8600 Rockville Pike, Bethesda, MD 20894
www.nlm.nih.gov

Wikipedia Encyclopedia
200 2nd Ave. South #358
St. Petersburg, FL 33701-4313
www.wikipedia.org

World Health Organization
www.who.int/en

About the Author

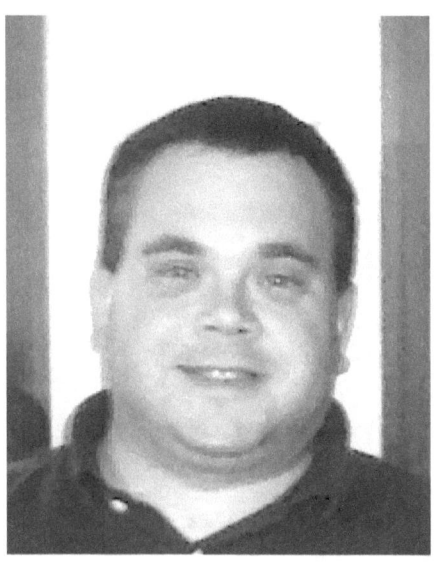

   The Author has led an interesting life. He has worked in a variety of fields ranging from Restaurant Management, Licensed Seaman, Educator, Journalist, and, is currently a Registered Nurse working in a Community Hospital nestled in the Adirondack Mountains. Academically he has earned a variety of degrees, which are listed in chronological order: AAA in Mass Media, BA in Communication Arts, AAS in Nursing, and finally a MS in Health Care Administration. He lives with his wife, Virginia, and their two sons, John and Seamus in the Adirondack Mountains in upstate New York.

www.ingramcontent.com/pod-product-compliance
Lightning Source LLC
Chambersburg PA
CBHW021302280526
45784CB00005B/2483